PERSPECTIVES IN BIOETHICS

POPE JOHN PAUL II LECTURE SERIES IN BIOETHICS

edited by

Rev. Francis J. Lescoe, Ph.D. and Rev. David Q. Liptak, D. Min.

. . . .

VOL. I
PERSPECTIVES IN BIOETHICS

I. CRITICAL REFLECTIONS ON CURRENT BIOETHICAL THINKING

by

Rev. Ronald D. Lawler, O.F.M., Cap., Ph.D.
Director, Center for Thomistic Studies, University of St. Thomas

II. "BEGOTTEN NOT MADE:" REFLECTIONS ON LABORATORY PRODUCTION OF HUMAN LIFE

by

William E. May, Ph.D.
Associate Professor of Theology, Catholic University of America

* * * *

INTRODUCTIONS

by

Most Rev. John F. Whealon, D.D., S.S.L., S.T.L.
Archbishop of Hartford

POPE JOHN PAUL II BIOETHICS CENTER
Holy Apostles College **Cromwell, Connecticut**

Library of Congress Catalog No. 83-06383

Lescoe, Francis J. and Liptak, David Q., Editors,
Pope John Paul II Lecture Series in Bioethics.
Vol. I
Lawler, Ronald D. and May, William E.,
Perspectives in Bioethics.

ISBN 0-910919-00-3

+ Daniel P. Reilly
Bishop of Norwich
September 16, 1982

Distributors for the trade:
MARIEL PUBLICATIONS
196 Eddy Glover Boulevard
New Britain, CT 06053

PRESIDENT'S MESSAGE

With deep gratitude, we thank Almighty God for enabling us at Holy Apostles College to establish the POPE JOHN PAUL II BIOETHICS CENTER.

Today's society is beset with crucial questions of morality and ethical values, springing from the fields of science, technology and medicine. Much time and dedication are needed for the safeguarding and promotion of basic principles, which will enable the faithful to form a right conscience, consonant with right reason and the official teachings of the Catholic Church.

Accordingly, we are most happy to announce that the students, staff, faculty and administrators of Holy Apostles College dedicate themselves to the fostering of the Church's official teaching in matters of faith and morals. This we propose to do through the inauguration of the POPE JOHN PAUL II LECTURE SERIES IN BIOETHICS.

Very Reverend Leo J. Ovian, M.Ss.A., Ph.D.
President-Rector

THE POPE JOHN PAUL II LECTURES
HAVE BEEN MADE POSSIBLE THROUGH
THE GENEROSITY OF
REVEREND LEO J. KINSELLA
AND
GENEVIEVE D. LUPA
OF
OUR LADY OF THE SNOWS PARISH
CHICAGO, ILLINOIS

TABLE OF CONTENTS

ANNOUNCEMENT

The Pope John Paul II Bioethics Center has been instituted for the purpose of articulating authentic Catholic teaching with respect to medical science and technology.

In his first encyclical, Redemptor Hominis, *John Paul defended the priority of ethics over science and technology:*

> *The development of technology and the development of contemporary civilization, which is marked by the ascendancy of technology, demand a proportional development of morals and ethics. (Section 16)*

Today, with an unprecedented rush of scientific discoveries and technological breakthroughs, this priority is being doubted, ignored and challenged. Traditional Christian principles repeatedly affirmed by the Church's magisterium have been set aside for consequentialism, behaviorism, relativism, context morality, secularism and other inadequate or erroneous theories in misleading, false and sometimes inane attempts to address ethically fresh scientific insights or revolutionary technological advances.

The purpose of this Center is twofold. First, we shall endeavor to impart to our seminarians, here at Holy Apostles College and Seminary, a solid foundation in medical ethics and bioethical science. Secondly, we shall share our investigations and findings by publishing periodic monographs, in addition to the annual Pope John Paul II Lectures in Bioethics.

INTRODUCTION OF FATHER RONALD LAWLER

by

Archbishop John F. Whealon

We are all aware that, in the 1980's, life has become unprecedently complicated. The most radical complications in our times concern issues of life and death, because they touch on the very meaning of life and of death. These current issues, all of them moral, run the gamut of human life: from the meaning and implications of conjugal love and the role of sex in marriage, to the question of how to treat the person who has reached the end of life's road, the terminally ill patient.

People committed to Jesus Christ, those dedicated to the defense of moral standards in our society *must* be fully informed on the scientific and legal aspects of the questions under discussion. The proponents of anti-life propositions – of artificial insemination, contraception, abortion, sterilization or euthanasia (to name a few of the volatile life issues) – know in detail the medical nature of each procedure and the latest court decision pertinent to the issue at hand. Those whe are dedicated to moral standards must be as familiar as their opponents with the precise nature and the morality of the acts under debate.

That is why the Lecture Series on Bioethics, sponsored by Holy Apostles College and Seminary, is so important for our times and for our area.

Personally and officially, I am delighted to present to you Father Ronald Lawler, a friend of many years who is fortunate indeed in his sibling. Father Lawler, a member of the 16th Century Catholic Franciscan Renewal Order of the Capuchins, received a doctorate in philosophy at St. Louis University and later studied philosophy and theology at Oxford University in England. He taught theology at Catholic University in Washington, and later taught and served as Dean of Theology at the Pontifical College Josephinum in Ohio. He was also the first President of the Fellowship of Catholic Scholars. Co-editor of *The Teaching of Christ* (for which I wrote), he now is Director of the

Center for Thomistic Studies at the University of St. Thomas in Houston, Texas.

Father Lawler speaks to us this evening on the topic *Critical Reflections on Current Bioethical Thinking*.

It is a privilege and pleasure to welcome to the Archdiocese of Hartford, and to present to you Father Ronald Lawler.

CRITICAL REFLECTIONS ON CURRENT BIOETHICAL THINKING

In the last two decades there has been an astonishing growth in the study of bioethics. It is an honor to be speaking here at the invitation of the Pope John Paul II Center for bioethical study. This is the newest of the many centers for study of bioethical questions in recent years.[1] Such centers reflect the abundant growth of research in these areas. Not only do we see today an increasing number of journals and newsletters devoted to moral questions touching medicine and other life sciences, but medical journals themselves are giving ever increasing attention to reflection on ethical issues. The huge bibliographies that appear in this field reflect the flood of books and articles being written.[2] Not only do schools of philosophy and theology now provide opportunities for advanced study in bioethics, but medical schools themselves are hiring ethicians and offering courses in unprecedented numbers.[3] It would be rash to say that we are more ethical in medicine today than our fathers were, but we do talk about ethics a lot more.

There are four points that I would like to make about this remarkable development in bioethical thinking. First, it was in a certain sense to be expected: it was and is necessary. Secondly, in another sense this development is surprising. The earnest discussion of ethical issues in live sciences is a blessing that we should seek to nourish. Third, the growth has of course not been entirely healthy. We live in a world of spiritual confusion: and word that Johnny or Mary is studying bioethics even in a Catholic high school or college is not necessarily good news. Finally, there is good reason to be optimistic about the future of bioethics.

I. BIOETHICS HAD TO GROW. The range of bioethics is wider than that of the medical ethics of old. Professor K. Danner Clouser speaks of it as extending to the whole bio-realm: not only to medicine, but to all the sciences and professions that touch life.[4] It would be concerned with environmental issues, with biological research into the new technologies of birth or studies in genetics; with fertility research and population studies. Clouser points out two reasons why bioethics had to grow. All these areas of study to which bioethics is applied have grown exponentially in the last decades. We have come to know a lot more, and are able to do a lot more, so that ethical questions that simply did not exist before have arisen before us and demand answers.[5] Moreover these questions in life sciences touch so closely the lives of all us that it would be inhuman not to think seriously about them.

Forty years ago we simply did not have the ways to ward off death that we now have. If a child were born with spina bifida he or she was likely to die. We could do no more than care for such children a little while. But now we have complex ways of saving their lives. In some cases, the lives we could save would be lives of much pain and would be severely limited; and sometimes great resources must be expended to save them. But since we can save them now we have a new question: ought we? And we must ask the question earnestly. In days of old, spouses who longed for children they did not have could resort to prayer; now they may resort to a great variety of techniques, technologies, and drugs. But about most of these there are serious new questions: is this a human and right way to initiate life? It used to be rather clear whether a person were dead or not, so that there was no room for a serious moral question: may this person rightly be considered as dead? Even King Lear in his madness could place a mirror at Cordelia's mouth, and know she was dead. But when machinery can keep vital signs flourishing, new ways of honestly detecting the coming of death are needed. Modern skill in organ transplantation created puzzling moral issues.

These new moral questions do not arise merely because people have fallen away from their old moral convictions: they arise because even familiar principles can be applied to new contexts and issues only with difficulty. One who firmly rejects abortion, or ever directly killing what is or probably is a human being, might yet wonder whether using DES (diethylstilbestrol) in the treatment of rape victims is moral or not: the question involves new complexities that need to be newly thought out.

II. SURPRISINGNESS OF THIS GROWTH. While growth in bioethics was necessary, we have reason to be both puzzled and pleased at the rise of a high tide of ethical interest in our day. University departments are having every kind of ethics course tailored these days: business ethics, engineering ethics, communications ethics, political ethics, and a further rich variety, along with bioethics.[6] Now in every case it can be said that the profound changes in every field have made such courses imperative—but it was not at all evident that they would actually come to be.

In fact, the dominant forms of ethical theory in English-speaking universities would tend to suggest that such professional ethics courses would *not* be established, and that the multiple centers of ethical inquiry would *not* be established.

A generation ago Alfred Jules Ayer in his essay "Critique of Ethics and Theology"[7] expressed in classical form the hostility of positivism to ethical thinking. He wrote: "It is plain that the conclusion that it is impossible to dispute questions of value follows from our theory also."[8] In Ayer's theory, "good" and "bad" are not genuine concepts with some definite assignable meaning. To say that abortion is wicked or that it is morally permissible would be equally meaningless utterances. Underlying moral statements are simply nonrational emotional attitudes. Some people happen to approve of abortion in some circumstances and some happen not to. Since moral judgments express attitudes and assert nothing rational, it would be ridiculous to try to prove a moral judgment true or false. Ayer argues further that people not only should not, but they cannot and do not ever "dispute about questions of value."[9] Ayer concedes that in a sense a person could have moral principles, that is, have an emotional stance that cause him to approve or disapprove various sorts of things. "What we do not and cannot argue about is the validity of these moral principles. We merely praise them or condemn them in light of our feelings."[10]

Ayer's theory is born out of his own version of logical positivism, a philosophy that was extremely popular especially before World War II. But it expresses a conviction that has long been common in the empiricist tradition: that we can establish the truth of matters of fact, but values cannot be known, proved or rationally debated.[11] Even when logical positivism faded, and contemporary forms of analytic philosophy arose, the conviction persisted that moral judgments about kinds of acts or about particular acts flow from chosen values, preferences, or commitments, and that it would be simply impossible to establish any one of them as actually true or false.[12]

For this reason ethics courses in this country in the main stream of analytic thought tended to ignore the great new questions that the rising technologies presented. If moral judgments about medical procedures are emotive utterances, if by their very logic and nature they cannot be true or false, it is not the work of a clear-headed thinker to try to establish the truth about them. That should be left to preachers, theologians and editorial writers, who are not thought (by philosophy professors) to be afflicted with clear analytic intelligence.[13] People may indeed have their preferences, and fight for them with all the rhetorical devices they can. But they should realize that there is no question here of determining the truth of the matter.

Many forms of popular moral education these days reflect this moral nihilism of positivism than they would care to acknowledge clearly. Many educators in value theory are bitterly opposed to what they call "indoctrination" especially because they really believe that nothing simply is morally good or bad, so that any teacher who bears witness to what he or she "knows" to be good or bad would be merely imposing a subjective opinion. Even some forms of education in Christian conscience are descendants of value scepticism. Each should follow his or her own conscience, because there can be no interpersonally valid knowledge of what is good or evil, even from a public divine revelation. If a person really judges something good or bad (often this becomes equivalent to really wanting to do or to avoid something), then it is good or bad for that person.[14]

Even when the dominant philosophy of an age is unable to explain the nature of moral judgments and moral debate, the need to face practical moral questions remains. In the sixties there was a great rebirth in interest in moral questions. People wanted not only to assert their convictions about war and sex and drugs and new technologies of death; they wanted to affirm that their convictions were right, and, even more, to insist that those who said otherwise were wrong.[15] It was not the mainstream professors of ethics who created the current concern for bioethics and other forms of professional ethics. Rather it was a great multitude of serious people who knew that changed conditions required decisions of them. They wished their decisions to be made intelligently, in ways that would authentically enrich their own lives and the lives of those they loved. They demanded ethics courses that would face the issues of the day. What they were seeking was a rational ordering of life, the very thing classical moralists always sought. Often they sought it in the midst of great spiritual disorder, themselves at times partly penetrated by the relativism and moral nihilism of the age, and at times penetrated by an earnest will to catch the truth of things in moral matters. That confusion weakens much moral debate today; but the earnestness that created profound concern for rational reflection on moral issues, even in quarters where philosophical resources to handle such questions well were drastically lacking, provides an opportunity that the Christian ethicist must delight in. If he has any good things to say, he has an audience disposed to listen.

III. NOT ALL IS WELL IN BIOETHICS. The Winter issue of *Listening: Journal of Religion and Culture* sounded a warning against taking too much pleasure in the current resurgence of interest in ethics. The editor of the issue, Professor Henry Veatch, noted that there is something puzzling about the contemporary eagerness to apply ethics to every kind of complex problem at a time when so many who do this are unwilling to recognize the literal truth of any principles that might be applied. "While, of course, no one is against ethics in these days—just as in former days no one was against things like God and motherhood—still might there not be ground for suspicion, when one is confronted with such a plethora of sudden attempted applications here, there and everywhere?"[16] For the most part, there is no effort to prove that any ethical principles are true (and there is a grave fear that any allegedly wise man who sought to communicate the truth of any moral judgment would be guilty of the sin of indoctrination.) Yet without knowing if our principles are true or not, we are eager to apply them to every kind of question. "And could not this indeed be the Achilles heel of all our new-fashioned, new-day ethics? Notice how in the Harvard Report nothing whatever is said about teaching students any *truths* of ethics; rather all the talk is about familiarizing students merely with 'ethical *problems*.' Or again, those educators who are so concerned with bringing ethics into the classroom have a way of always sliding away from the question of whether ethics is an affair of genuine knowledge, and hence the kind of thing that can legitimately be taught. Instead, the emphasis is all on the kind of thing often called 'values clarification' — as if the concern in ethics education, so called, were simply to acquaint students with what might be called values alternatives, it then being up to the students 'to make up their own minds' just which of the assorted sets of values they would opt for, each of them for themselves."[17]

All this is a besetting temptation of the times. People want to know what it would be right and wise to do; but they don't want to grasp a truth so lucid that they might feel actually required to walk in its light. The great moral philosophers of the ages, Plato, Aristotle, Augustine, Aquinas, Kierkegaard, passionately sought what was truly good. They realized that the quest for moral truth was especially difficult. One must seek the truly good with all one's heart and energy. The wise man did not take the stance of a cynic, reluctant to be forced to acknowledge moral truth. Neither would he affirm them mindlessly. But with all one's resources, with integrity and care, the truth of how to lead a wise and good life is to be sought.[18]

I do not wish to take here the role of the pessimist. Many good things are happening in contemporary ethics. But Veatch has certainly touched an important point. In the same issue of *Listening* I had contributed an article with the somewhat cynical title: "Professional Ethics Courses: Do They Corrupt the Young?"[19] My own answer was that they very easily can, though they need not. Certainly I hope I am not corrupting the young people among you as I speak of bioethics here. But a study of some of the more popular textbooks in metaethics shows rather clearly how demoralizing study of them could be.[20]

Usually a contemporary textbook will begin with an introductory section on moral theory, in which different positions on basic issues are sketched. There will be a brief treatment of what morality means to the utilitarian or consequentialist; sadly, this will often be labeled (with total disregard for what teleology meant in classical ethics) "teleological" thinking. Often there will be a treatment of some Kantian form of thinking; this will be labeled "deontological." Other forms of moral theory will be noted: perhaps cultural relativism and subjectivism; and there may be some explicit discussion of noncognitivism. Normally there will be no effort to urge that any of these theories is true. One is to look over the advantages and disadvantages of each, not with the hunger and thirst for moral truth of a Kierkegaard or an Augustine, but with the polite detachment of Newman's unfortunate gentleman. It would be gauche to seek truth here too passionately; to teach as though one had found a truth that he loved to share with another would be to flirt with the severe sin of indoctrination. The result of all this dispassionate treatment is predictable.[21] The intelligent student realizes that he is not going to learn whether any of these broad views is or could be decisively true. So he wishes to rush into the "real questions," where hopefully something definite can be decided.

Alas, the hope is rather desperate. When difficult contemporary questions are raised, the situation becomes really hopeless. Their textbooks are anthologies of articles written with considerable dialectical skill in defense of sharply opposed positions. The arguments in different articles are extremely difficult to assess. Authors appeal to different kinds of evidence; they have different presuppositions about the proper forms of moral argumentation. Each is soliciting the reader's approval for reasons that it would be difficult to analyze and reduce to principles; but if the student could reduce them to principles, it would not help him, for he has not been helped to get personal possession of or insight into the validity of any particular principles anyway. Hence the student becomes more and more convinced that he cannot really give intelligent answers to moral questions. He can only take sides, hoping that he has guessed rightly about good and evil. Nothing could seem better calculated to lead one from the earnest hope that first lead to the study of ethics: the hunger to know what is really good, the form of life actually worth living.

Hence, precious as the new interest in bioethics is, it can have unhappy consequences for many. Often young medical students approach the study of bioethics already in possession of some moral convictions that they realize are true, although the mode with which they grasp them is not scientific or clear. Both the Greek and Judaeo-Christian traditions held that it is very possible to possess with certainty true moral positions before one enrolls in an ethics course.[22] Greek philosophers, in fact, tended to believe that the seeds of virtue had to be planted (by wise teachers: i.e., by those who *knew* something of good and evil) and by living among virtuous people, so that one came to know what is truly good by tasting what is truly good in virtuous action. Students often approach ethics courses hoping that these courses will reveal to them the roots and grounds of their deepest hopes and convictions. Unfortunately in badly taught courses they can become convinced that what they have known is not knowable; so that their last state is worse than the first.

When people become convinced that no particular position can be known to be noble and right, they can drift toward inhuman ethical positions. The contemporary bioethical world at times speaks of a new ethics that is about to overtake the old ethics. The supposedly "old" ethics, that of classical positions of virtue and natural law, that of a religious view of truly good ways made known by divine revelation and intelligent understanding, is to be replaced by a self-styled "new" ethic: relativistic, without recognition of inalienable human rights in each person, consequentialist, ready to do evil if good will come of it. This new ethics is openly embraced by many. A much-quoted editorial in the journal *California Medicine* declares that the new ethic will be a relativistic one. No longer will we define "the intrinsic worth and equal value of every human life regardless of its stage or condition."[23] Already, the journal argues, "we" have ceased believing that. The needs of the time have driven us to place only relative value on individual human lives. If the quality of many lives can be improved by killing some human beings, we will want to do that; and we will; and we will create an ethics to justify it. In fact, we do this already. The article (clearly it supports abortion) forthrightly acknowledges that an abortion is the killing of a human being. When some pro-abortionists deny "the scientific fact, which everyone really knows, that human life begins at conception and is continuous, whether intra- or extra-uterine until death,"[24] the reason for this curious denial is that they have not yet shaken off the hangups of the old ethic. They still feel that each human being should be treated as an end, not as a means. But they also feel (and this more strongly) that they want intensely to achieve their own longed for goals, and they wish to have them even if other human beings must suffer for it. Until they get courage to affirm boldly the new ethics, they must pretend they are not acting against the values of the old ethic that they clearly are acting against.

Such brazen anti-personalist stands can be found in the bioethical literature of our time. In fact, very many well known bioethicians defend views that assail the dignity of human persons. There are very many defenders of abortion, and growing numbers who would justify infanticide and euthanasia.[25] Despite the tragic experience with human experimentation by Nazi physicians, some bioethicians take intolerably casual attitudes toward experimentation on humans without informed consent. [26] Those who indoctrinate young people in relativistic consequentialism insist that they are not indoctrinating when they are trying to prove their principles, and so argue that no specific moral principles are always valid. Indoctrinating is what principled moralists do when they try to prove their principles.

IV. GOOD REASONS FOR HOPE. But it would be absurd and demoralizing to suggest that entry into the world of contemporary bioethics is entry into a world simply dominated by relativism, consequentialism, rejection of the humane and insistent principles that have protected human dignity through the centuries. Nor should Catholic people, who often have reasons for a special anxiety about theologians who probe such issues, feel excessive concern. There have, indeed, been a number of moral thinkers in the Church, treating a variety of bioethical questions, who have conspicuously rejected the magisterial teaching of the Church. Some of them have been so honored by dissenting associates and by the media that a vague impression arises that these are the great and creative moralists of the day. But this is far from the truth. The great Catholic ethicians of the day are hardly those lionized by the *National Catholic Reporter*. If one were to seek the two English-speaking Catholic moralists today who are most respected throughout the world, by secular as well as religious thinkers, they would almost certainly be Elizabeth Anscombe, who holds the chair of

Philosophy at Cambridge University, and John Finnis, of Oxford.[27] Interestingly, each of these (like the majority of Catholic moralists working today) is a moralist whose thought is fully in accord with authentic Catholic teaching, personalistic, defending the human rights with clear teachings on moral absolutes, and successful in making peace between the received moral teaching of the western tradition and the legitimate needs of a contemporary expression of morality. As the Pope John Paul II Center for bioethics engages in moral research, it has no lack of great Catholic moral thinkers upon whom it can draw with confidence: creative and principled moralists like Germain Grisez, Vernon Bourke, Ralph McInerny, William May, Joseph Boyle.[28] And there is a wide range of non-catholic moralists, including the most creative among today's bioethical experts, whose fundamental principles are deeply in accord with the personalistic ethics of Catholicism. One need mention only a few names: Paul Ramsey, Arthur Dyck, Basil Mitchell, Stanley Hauerwas, Fred Carney. Should any wish to lament that the whole world has run off toward consequentialism and relativism, he would have to ignore the most intelligent and influential moralists of our time. The days are not bad ones for authentic Christian and personalistic ethics of a principled kind.

But there is one contemporary moralist who can most of all give heart to the creative ethician today. Certainly it is a singular blessing that in this time of tension and of opportunity in moral thinking that a distinguished Catholic moralist should have been elected pope. John Paul II had many scholarly interests; but his fundamental work over these last thirty years has been that of the ethician. He has studied the living questions of our time long and with great care, and has been in dialogue with the great minds of the times, teaching and lecturing not only in Poland, but throughout the world community. His election brought a remedy to a problem many had felt. The pope and bishops had been teaching one vision in moral thought; certain celebrated moralists were teaching another. The division between witnessing to faith and the insights of scholarship had to be bridged. Some feared that Church officials simply did not understand why the moralists were crying out for a change in standard teachings. But this pope clearly understands. And we have seldom had pastoral leaders with so much pastoral compassion. In him we have a new sign of hope and unity.[29]

Like other great Catholic moralists of the time, John Paul has studied carefully the differences between the two kinds of thinking dominant in the world today. Consequentialist thinking is concerned with results: it is not so important what people do, i.e., what the actions that make up their lives *are*. What is significant will be the effects of their actions, what they bring about in the obscurities of this contingent world. The principled moralist, on the other hand, holds with the whole Catholic tradition that the actions one performs, the life one lives, is far more important than the consequences that may follow as physical consequences of these actions.[30] The logic of consequentialism is one that rejects absolutes: for a proportionate reason, one would be justified in doing the sorts of acts that authentic teaching always called instrinsically wrong. But principled thinking holds that men have inalienable rights, rights that may be violated for no proportionate reason whatever; that there are absolute duties, not in order to oppress men, but to guard authentic values and the dignity of each person.

John Paul's position on this question is very clear. "The human act is simultaneously transitive and non-transitive. It is transitive inasmuch as it goes to the other side of the subject, seeking an expression or an effect in the external world, and thus objectivises itself in some product. It is non-transitive in the measure in which 'remaining in the subject' in which it determines the quality and the value, and establishes his own 'fieri' essentially human. Therefore man, in acting not only fulfills some action, but in some way realizes himself, becomes himself."[31]

That is to say, human actions cause effects in the world. But they also cause effects in the depths of the human person. The more profound and important effect is that which a human action has on the person himself. Our actions are our lives. When we choose to do the actions we do, we choose to make ourselves the kinds of persons who do such things. We create ourselves, and show the direction in which our heart is willing and desires to go.

When, even in tragic cases, one does a deed that is in itself simply a doing of evil (for example, starving to death a baby who is considered defective, or killing an aged and suffering person) in the hope that something good may come of it, then one is taking a view of the world very different from that which shaped the judgment of the saints. It is a view that producing good effects, having fine things *happen* in the world, is better and more important than *doing* actions which are free deeds honoring God by their goodness; and that having painful things happen is worse than having free persons deliberately doing deeds which are unequivocally attacks on real goods in real persons.[32] At heart consequentialism is the view that the prime way of loving persons is that of making this world a pleasant and happy place; while the saints felt that the world is a place in which souls are made, in which persons are shaped by their own free actions. The most important thing that anyone can do is to do excellent and good deeds, not out of self-love or in a desire to esteem oneself for one's "virtue," but rather because one recognizes that the person as an image of God serves his brothers and sisters by pursuing only good in his life, pursuing it well, and never doing evil that good may come of it, never treating what is good in any person or personal act as if it were evil.

Medical ethics has gone astray most severely when it sought to justify doing bad kinds of deeds for excellent reasons. The most shocking pages in medical history flow from such decisions. Nazi doctors did not engage in human experimentation of cruel kinds simply to be cruel; they hoped to accomplish important goals useful for humanity by such vicious behavior. Now it is true that we have a duty to make this world a good place, to care about the consequences of our conduct. But we must care first of all about what we do, about the actions that are our life; and seek always to achieve good only by good means.

In treating one bioethical question in his Apostolic Exhortation *Familiaris Consortio,* Pope John adverts to the very different conclusions than a principled and a consequentialistic mode of thinking may come to in this matter. And he noted with a certain intensity that the difference between the two views "is much wider and deeper than is usually thought, one which involves in the final analysis two irreconcilable concepts of the human person."[33] To adopt the principled view of morality that one must never, for any reason, attack any basic good in any person is to adopt the view that every person is of transcendent dignity; it is to treat all men as images of God. To adopt the view that one may attack basic goods in a person when there is a proportionate reason is to judge that in the end human beings may be treated as means serving the purposes of others.[34]

One schooled in the paths of Christian wisdom will not do deeds that are direct attacks on any authentic good in any person in the vain hope of making the world better by such deeds. Whether the material world and the circumstances of human living will be better or worse in the future, we cannot know with certainty. We are uncertain of the effects of even our best intended actions. What we are sure of is that if we do acts that are faithful to the dignity of every person, and honor every human value in every person, then we will be honoring God in our life, and he who is the absolute ruler of providence will be able to make of all our labors something that serves the growth of the kingdom. St. Thomas More tried in every honorable way to save his life that he might participate more richly in goods that he loved on earth. But he was right in judging that it would be wrong to participate in every kind of good by means of doing an act which was itself wrong.[35] The reason for this is not that rules are to be more honored than persons, but that persons and human actions, what people *do,* and what they *are* is more important than what happens to them. The transient effects of our actions on the world and on persons can, as every medical professional and every intelligent person well knows, be frighteningly important. But in this world of persons, nothing is more important for the good of each and of all, than the excellence of the actions that are the core of our lives.

What modes of thinking and teaching and living will dominate in the world of bioethics in the years immediately before us? The answer is not predetermined: it lies in our own hands. The medical and life professions are surely tempted to yield to the blandishments of a "new" ethic—an ethic essentially like that of the pre-Socratics, who, having despaired of the possibility of coming to know what is absolutely good, encouraged their disciples instead to do what they earnestly wanted to do as though they did not know the dark depths of the human spirit when it despairs of knowing what is authentically good, and deserving of full loyalty. But the medical and life professions are tempted too by that newer and richer ethic of the Golden Age of Greece, and of the Enlightenment, and especially of the fire of the Judaeo-Christian visions—that ethics of personal rights, and principles that endure, and values that are good beyond measure—that ethic that requires self-discipline, yet gives freedom and dignity to the human spirit.

In recent years I have taught bioethics in a great many contexts: in secular and religious universities, to medical students, to seminarians. Obviously young people of our time feel the pressures of the age toward moral solutions which are convenient, but do not respect every person and every basic human value. But it has seemed to me that when the young people of our time begin to understand what is at stake, and what it is that they themselves want in their own lives, that they have almost universally chosen gladly to adopt that form of moral thinking that defends the dignity of the person more securely. The future is full of hope if we give our young people a real opportunity to lay hold of the moral heritage they have a right to know well. But it will remain necessary to help them see how the bracing principles of Christian morality are not exercises in legalism, but protections of the freedom and dignity of the human person.

NOTES

1. Major centers for the study of bioethics in this country include The Hastings Center (Institute of Society, Ethics, and the Life Sciences), Hasting-on-Hudson, New York; The Pope John XXIII Medical-Moral Research Center, St. Louis, Missouri and The Kennedy Center for the Study of Human Reproduction and Bioethics, Georgetown University, Washington, D.C.. Like the second of these, the Pope John Paul II Center, Cromwell, Connecticut, is concerned to study bioethical questions in the light of the moral teaching of the Catholic Church.
2. Useful and relatively complete continuing bibliographies include the *Bibliography of Society, Ethics, and the Life Sciences,* published by the Hastings Center; Walter Leroy, ed., *Bibliography of Bioethics* (Detroit: Gale Publishing Co., 1975 -   ) (a large volume is published each year in this series). The *Encyclopedia of Bioethics* (New York: Free Press, 1978) is also an exceptionally good source for helpful bibliographies.
3. For a study of the growth of the study of bioethics, see R. Veatch, W. Gaylin, and C. Morgan, eds., *The Teaching of Medical Ethics* (Hastings-on-Hudson, N.Y.: Hastings Center, 1973). For a survey of the history of medical ethics and education in medical ethics, see the series of articles in the *Encyclopedia of Bioethics,* vol. 3 and 4, pp. 870-1007.
4. K.D. Clouser, "Bioethics," in *Encyclopedia of Bioethics,* vol. 1, p. 120.
5. *Op. cit.,* pp. 124-25.
6. See Henry Veatch, "Ethics and Applied Ethics: an Introductory Note," *Listening* XVII (Winter, 1982), pp. 3-6.
7. This essay is the sixth chapter of A.J. Ayer, *Logic, Truth, and Language* (Oxford: Oxford University Press, 1936). The second edition of this work has an important new preface (1946) modifying the militancy of the first edition's severe positivism.
8. *Op. cit.,* p. 110.
9. *Ibid.*
10. *Op cit.,* pp. 111-12.
11. This familiar position, that all values are based on subjective evaluations, so that nothing at all can be strictly and objectively *known* to be good or bad, is expressed, e.g., in R.B. Perry, *General Theory of Value* (Cambridge: Harvard University Press, 1926); it has been a common position among liberal behavioral scientists.
12. This conclusion is defended by many, such as Professor R.M. Hare, of Oxford, because of a strange conviction that the kind of freedom required by morality demands that each person must freely choose his or her own moral principle (i.e., cannot possibly discover that any are true, and worthy of being freely chosen for that reason.) For these moralists no principle could be simply true and morally binding for anyone before one chose to commit oneself in a certain way. See Hare, *The Language of Morals* (Oxford: Clarendon, 1963). p. 60 ff. See also the critique of this position by R. Lawler, *Philosophical Analysis and Ethics* (Milwaukee: Bruce, 1968), pp. 95-109.

13. Cf., e.g., C.L. Stevenson, *Ethics and Language* (New Haven: Yale University Press, 1955), ch. 1 and ch. 11.
14. For a critique of these positions, see Paul C. Vitz, " 'Values Clarification' in the Schools," *New Oxford Review,* June 1981, pp. 15-20, and "Secular Humanism and Morality," *New Oxford Review,* July-August 1981, pp. 12-126. See also Paul Philibert, "Moral Education and the Formation of Conscience," and William B. Smith, "The Meaning of Conscience," both in William May, ed., *Principles of Catholic Moral Life* (Chicago: Franciscan Herald Press, 1981), pp. 383-411 and 361-382.
15. This point was stressed by Julian Huxley in his critique of Nazi ethics in "Evolutionary Ethics," The Romanes Lectures, 1943, in T.H. Huxley and J. Huxley, *Touchstone for Ethics* (New York: Harper, 1947), p. 114.
16. Henry Veatch, *op. cit.,* p. 14.
17. *Op. cit.,* pp. 14-15.
18. Thus Socrates, Plato, and Aristotle were passionately concerned to transcend the shadowy opinions that the Sophists dealt with, to examine life with depth and to pursue the real truth of things, to grasp what is actually good, what makes life actually worth living.
19. R. Lawler, "Professional Ethics Courses: Do They Corrupt the Young?", *Listening* (Winter, 1982), pp. 7-17.
20. Granted their own ground rules, some of these studies are well-constructed indeed. Their surveys of ethical theories are conscientiously done (though they reveal no passion to pursue what might really be true in such matters), and the collections of essays on specific questions are, in some cases, very well chosen. Among the best books of this kind one might note: S. Gorowitz et al., eds., *Moral Problems in Medicine* (Englewood Cliffs, N.J.: Prentice-Hall, 1979), and L. Beauchamp and L. Walters, eds., *Moral Problems in Medicine* (Encino, Calif.: Dickenson, 1977).
21. John Henry Newman's reflections on this point remain instructive. See *The Idea of a University* (London: Longmans, Green, 1947) (originally published 1852), Lecture VIII.
22. Thus the *Republic* of Plato reflected a Greek conviction that one could come to a personal knowledge of what is good only if one were educated in ways that led to virtue; but that the virtuous man can in fact come to a knowledge of what is good. Christian philosophies had many ways of teaching that young people need to be formed in excellent ways of living before they will be able to grasp intellectually the ultimate roots of the excellence of these ways; but that coming to true intellectual insight into these matters is possible.
23. An Editorial, "A New Ethics for Medicine and Society," in *California Medicine,* September 1970, reprinted in R. Baum, ed., *Ethical Arguments for Analysis* (New York: Holt, Rinehart, and Winston, 1976), p. 186.
24. *Ibid.*
25. Cf. e.g., Michael Tooley, "Infanticide and Abortion," *Philosophy and Public Affairs* 2 (1973) pp. 37-65.
26. For an introduction to this question, see Paul Ramsey, *The Patient*

as Person (New Haven: Yale University Press, 1970), pp. 1-58; see also K. Lebacqz and R. Levine, "Informed Consent: Ethical and Moral Aspects,"*Encyclopedia of Bioethics*, vol. II, pp. 754-62.

27. G.E.M. Anscombe is Professor of Philosophy at Cambridge University. Her collected works have recently been published by the University of Minnesota Press: G.E.M. Anscombe, *Collected Philosophical Papers* (Minneapolis: University of Minnesota Press, 1981), 3 vol. John M. Finnis is Praelector in Jurisprudence and University College and Reader in Law, University of Oxford. He has recently published *Natural Law and Natural Rights* (Oxford: Clarendon Press, 1980), the tenth volume in the distinguished Clarendon Law Series. Anscombe and Finnis are certainly, in the eyes of the secular intellectual community, the most respected of Catholic moral theorists. Even more creative is the work of Germain Grisez, professor of moral theology at Mt. St. Mary's Seminary, Emmitsburg, Md. Grisez is now preparing a striking new moral synthesis in moral theology that is far more inclusive and innovative than the work of any of the prominent dissenters, yet entirely faithful to received Catholic teaching. See especially his *Christian Moral Principles,* Second Draft, a privately printed preliminary edition (Emmitsburg, Md.: Mount Saint Mary's Seminary, 1981). This is a preparatory edition of the first volume of a projected four volume study of Catholic moral theology.
28. We use the term "principled" in contrast with "consequentialist." In this distinction, the principle moralist holds that there are some principles which are known to be universally true, from which, in reflection on relevant facts, one can deduce true, certain, and exceptionless conclusions in some ethical questions. Consequentialists generally hold that there are no moral principles with specific though universal content that are known to be universally true. Thus for them slaying the wicked may be said to be generally wicked, but one would be justified in doing such a deed in a particular case if one had a proportionate reason for so doing. Some comments on consequentialism will be given below.
29. Before his election to the papacy as John Paul II. Karol Wojtyla published many important works in moral theory and its application to contemporary problems. See especially his *Love and Responsibility* (New York: Farrar, Straus, Giroux, 1981). For his critique of consequentialism (utilitarianism) in this work, see pp. 34-39.
30. See John Paul II's treatment of this point in his *Encyclical Letter* "Laborem Exercens" (September 14, 1981), nn. 6 - 9.
31. Karol Wojtyla, *Ocena mozliwosci,* p. 122; cited in A. Woznicki, *Karol Wojtyla's Existential Personalism* (New Britain, Ct.: Mariel, 1979), p. 47. See also R. Lawler, *The Christian Personalism of John Paul II* (Chicago: Franciscan Herald Press, 1982), pp. 51-74.
32. The contrast between the mode of thinking in scholarly saints like Thomas More and the positions of consequentialists is hard to exaggerate. Thomas More was utterly opposed to swearing falsely, even to save his own life, to save his wife and children, to provide the King with good counsellors, and the like. Calculation did not

enter into such questions: faithfulness to true and enduring principles, to the goodness of truth and the duty never to act directly against it, were decisive, whatever the consequences. In defense of the position that one may properly act directly against great human goods for a proportionate reason, Richard McCormick expresses his belief that those who are unwilling to act directly against a great human good in some person for the sake of some other good probably do not love the good not acted for as do those who would willingly act directly against the basic good in question. See R. McCormick, *Ambiquity in Moral Choice* (Milwaukee: Marquette University Press, 1977), p. 88. Apply this to the situation in Thomas More's time: did those Englishmen who were willing to swear falsely, as Thomas was not, in order to care for their wives and children, and obtain other goals, really have a more intense love for their wives and children than Thomas More had for his? It would be an absurdity to pretend that; cf. his letters to his daughter, and the studies of contemporary biographers. Thomas More loved intensely the goods he was to lose because he was faithful to the truth; but nothing could lead him to attack basic values like truth and loyalty to the faith. See E.E. Reynolds, *The Life and Death of Thomas More,* esp. chs. 27 and 28.

33. John Paul II. *Apostolic Exhortation* "Familiaris Consortio," (November 22, 1981), n. 32.
34. See the comments of Bernard Williams, of Cambridge University, on the demoralizing fruits of consequentialist thinking in J.J. Smart and B. Williams, *Utilitariansim: For and Against* (London: Cambridge University Press, 1973, esp. pp. 108-34. See also J. Finnis, *Natural Law and Natural Rights,* pp. 111-25, and G. Grisez, "Against Consequentialism," *American Journal of Jurisprudence* 23 (1978) pp. 21-38.
35. The playwright Robert Bolt catches the spirit of More's principled thinking, his firm refusal to do the evil and self-destroying deed of swearing falsely for any reason whatever, throughout his *A Man for All Seasons* (New York: Random House, 1960).

INTRODUCTION OF DR. WILLIAM MAY
by
Archbishop John F. Whealon

The past twenty years – the fascinating two decades since the start of the Second Vatican Council – have been the era of *aggiornamento*. During this period of the Church's history, all teachings and traditions of the Catholic Church have been, as it were, taken out of their wrappings and inspected minutely to check their relevance in the modern world.

Aggiornamento makes sense for a Catholic only when a person knows that the divine element in the Church and its teachings cannot be changed. The human element – the accidentals, the style, the vocabulary – these are features that in *aggiornamento* can and should be updated. This Conciliar program is to make the eternal, unchanging truths of the faith more intelligible and acceptable to people of this age.

During the past twenty years the one area of Church doctrine that has fared worst under *aggiornamento* has been moral theology. In this one discipline the challenges have been most difficult. Those challenges have been to remain faithful to God's Revelation, to our Catholic tradition, to the magisterium so basic to Catholic Christianity – and at the same time to confront the new existential modes of thought as well as the ancient enemies of Christian ethics: the world, the flesh and the devil.

Our speaker this evening, Dr. William May, has been one of the few skillful enough to steer his craft carefully between Scylla and Charybdis during these past years. Doctor May, a Catholic layman, is Associate Professor of Moral Theology at the Catholic University of America. He has served as editor of the Newman Press and Bruce Publishing Company, has edited and authored articles and books almost past counting, and more basically has been an active layman in his parish and diocese.

I salute him especially for his valued work as chief consultant to the U.S. Bishops on their 1976 Pastoral

Letter, *To Live in Christ Jesus*. This, one of the best if not the best moral teaching ever given by the U.S. Bishops, was quoted repeatedly by Pope John Paul II when he visited our nation in 1979.

Tonight we hear the second lecture in a series of lectures named for Pope John Paul II. To the host institution, St. Thomas Seminary, and to the sponsoring institution, Holy Apostles College, I voice the gratitude of the local Church for making possible this timely lecture in bioethics. These are the new questions that now confront the Church in the modern world, relating to the meaning of life and origins of human life itself.

With pleasure, I introduce Dr. William May, speaking on *"Begotten Not Made": Reflections on the Generation of Human Life*.

"Begotten, Not Made": Reflections on the Laboratory Generation of Human Life

July 25, 1978, is a memorable date. First of all, it marked the tenth anniversary of Pope Paul VI's encyclical on marriage, *Humanae Vitae,* in which he affirmed that there is an indissoluble union willed by God and not to be deliberately sundered by human choice between the unitive or love-giving and the procreative or life-giving meanings of human sexuality.[1] The significance of Pope Paul's claim for assessing the laboratory generation of human life will be a central concern of this paper. This date is further notable in that it is the birthday of Louise Brown, the "test tube" baby, the miracle child of modern technology. Louise was the first baby to be born after having been conceived outside her mother's body by a process known as in vitro fertilization.

In vitro fertilization is the name given to the act of generating human life in the laboratory by fertilizing a human ovum, taken from the body of a woman by a procedure called laparoscopy, with human sperm provided by a male. The being brought into existence by this process is nurtured at first in the laboratory until it reaches the stage of development when it can be implanted in a human womb, where, it is hoped, it will undergo intrauterine development until normal birth.

In Louise Brown's case the same woman provided the ovum and subsequently nurtured in her womb the developing human life and, after birth, continues to act as Louise's mother. Moreover the sperm used to fertilize Mrs. Brown's ovum was provided by her husband. Still various permutations and combinations of in vitro fertilization are possible. Thus different women could (a) provide the ovum, (b) nurture the developing human life within the womb, and (c) act as the sociological mother of the child after birth; and the sperm could be provided by a male other than the spouse of the woman from whom the ovum is taken or the woman(en) who would bear and/or raise the child. In order to focus attention on what I believe is *the* central issue raised by the laboratory generation of human life, however, I shall limit consideration to the use of in vitro fertilization by married couples, with the wife nurturing the child in her own womb, the husband providing the sperm, and both carrying out parental responsibilities to the child given existence by this process.

In vitro fertilization is not the only form of the laboratory generation of human life possible. One that is theoretically possible, although it has not thus far been successfully attempted with human life, is nuclear transplantation or cloning, a completely asexual mode of reproduction inasmuch as it does not require the union of male and female gametes. In cloning, the nucleus of an unfertilized ovum is destroyed by radiation and is then replaced by the nucleus of a somatic cell taken from some human person's body. The ovum will then have a full set of chromosomes and will begin to develop as if it had been fertilized by a sperm, and it will develop, moreover, as an identical twin of the person whose somatic cell supplied the nucleus that was transplanted into the denucleated ovum.[2] Although cloning is, therefore, a possible form of the laboratory generation of human life, I will in what follows prescind from a consideration of this procedure insofar as what I will have to say about in vitro fertilization will be applicable *a fortiori* to cloning.

In addition to in vitro fertilization and cloning, in which human life is generated in the laboratory and not within the body of a human female, there is another form of "artful childmaking" already widely employed in our culture, that separates the generation of human life from the act of marital coition and that involves the participation, in generating life, of a person or persons other than the married couple. This form of artful childmaking is artificial insemination, of which there are two principal modes. In the first, called heterologous or "vendor"[3] insemination, the sperm that fertilizes the ovum within the body of the woman is provided by a male other than her husband. In the second, termed homologous insemination or artificial insemination by the husband, the sperm fertilizing the ovum is provided by the husband of the woman whose ovum is fertilized. Since artificial insemination of either modality is not, strictly speaking, a form of generating human life in the laboratory, I shall also prescind in what follows from a consideration of this form of artful child-making, and in particular, from an explicit reflection on a very serious issue raised by heterologous or vendor insemination, namely, the choice by a married woman to share her power of generating human life with a person other than her husband. Nonetheless, as will become evident, reflective analysis of in vitro fertilization involving a married couple will force us to come to terms with the key moral issue raised not only by the laboratory generation of human life but by all forms of artful childmaking that include the choice to separate the generation of human life from the act of marital coition.

What I shall now do is the following: (1) present the purposes that in vitro fertilization may serve for married persons; (2) discuss the major arguments used to justify in vitro fertilization for these purposes and, in the course of presenting them, note one of the most serious objections that has been advanced to oppose this practice; and (3) develop what I believe is the definitive reason why in vitro fertilization and all other modes of generating human life outside of the marital act are not morally worthy of human choice.

1. *Purposes of In Vitro Fertilization for Married Couples*

Richard A. McCormick, the eminent Jesuit theologian who is currently Rose F. Kennedy Professor of Christian Ethics at Georgetown University's Kennedy Center for Bioethics, has noted that there are two generic purposes that "reproductive interventions" such as in vitro fertilization might serve. The first he calls individual or personal purposes, and by this he means that a reproductive intervention such as in vitro fertilization will enable a couple childless because of some physical anomaly to have a child of their own. Thus in the case of Louise Brown and in other subsequently recorded cases of children brought to birth after in vitro fertilization the purpose of in vitro fertilization was to alleviate the couple's infertility caused by blocked fallopian tubes in the mother. The second generic purpose McCormick noted is eugenic, either positive or negative.[4] Although a few scientists have championed the use of reproductive interventions including in vitro fertilization for positive eugenic purposes, McCormick pointed out that the majority of scientists reject this possiblility as utterly unworkable and even dangerous.[5] He did not, however, comment at any length on the possible negative eugenic purposes that in vitro fertilization might serve. Therefore I would like to suggest some. Although these are not today technically feasible, I do not think that they are in principle unworkable and that they may, given sufficient technological advancement, be feasible in the future.

We know, for example, that a married couple, each of whom is the bearer of some recessive genetic defect such as Tay-Sachs disease, runs a twenty-five percent risk of having a child who will actually be crippled by this terrible disease should they choose to generate life through the marital act. It may perhaps be possible to remove ova, examine them to determine whether they bear the genes responsible for the disease in question or not, destroy those that do bear these genes, and then fertilize in vitro an ovum that does not carry these genes with her husband's sperm, implanting the developing fetus in her womb where it can then develop until birth. A child generated in this way would definitely not run the risk of being afflicted with the genetically induced disease, although he or she might, like his or her parents, be a carrier of the disease should the sperm used to fertilize the ovum bear the genes in question. Should it be possible to identify sperm as well as ova carrying the genes responsible for the disease and separate them from sperm that are free of such genes, it would then be possible to generate a child not only free from the disease but not even the carrier of genes responsible for causing it. Although it is definitely not possible today to use in vitro fertilization for this purpose—to help a couple known to be carriers of a crippling genetic disorder have a child free of risk of being afflicted with it—this may be feasible in the future. Were it to become so, resort to in vitro fertilization would surely be a more appropriate and humane way of coping with the problem than are the proposals that are currently made, namely, to have such couples generate life through the marital act, perform an amniocentesis at an advanced stage of pregnancy, and then abort should this procedure show that the developing human life is in all likelihood afflicted with the genetic malady,[6] or else have the wife inseminated by sperm provided by a vendor who is not himself the carrier of the recessive genes in question.[7]

2. *Arguments to Justify the Use of In Vitro Fertilization for Married Couples*

Here I will examine the major arguments advanced to support the use of in vitro fertilization, particularly as a way of helping married couples have a child of their own, couples who otherwise could not. There are two major sorts of arguments: one that in principle justifies not only in vitro fertilization as a way of alleviating the heartfelt desire of a married couple, otherwise childless, to have a child of their own, but also other types of artful childmaking, including in vitro fertilization by nonmarried persons, vendor insemination, and so forth; the second is more cautious and is intended in principle to justify exclusively the use of in vitro fertilization to help a married couple, otherwise childless, to have a child of their own.

The first sort of argument is advanced by such authors as Joseph Fletcher, Robert Francoeur, and Michael Hamilton.[8] The form in which this argument is cast by Joseph Fletcher merits attention, both because it summarizes briefly the type of reasoning employed by all who welcome the advent of the laboratory generation of human life and because in it we can discern the principal presuppositions behind the reasoning employed. Fletcher argues as follows:

> Man is a maker and a selector and a designer, and the more rationally contrived and deliberate anything is, the more human it is. Any attempt to set up an antinomy between

> natural and biological reproduction, on the one hand, amd artificial or designed reproduction, on the other, is absurd. The real difference is between accidental or random reproduction and rationally willed or chosen reproduction . . . If it [the latter] is "unnatural" it can only be so in the sense that all medicine is . . . It seems to me that laboratory reproduction is radically human compared to conception by ordinary heterosexual intercourse. It is willed, chosen, purposed, and controlled, and surely these are among the traits that distinguish *homo sapiens* from others in the animal genus . . . Genital reproduction is, therefore, less human than laboratory reproduction, more fun, to be sure, but with our separation of baby making from love making, both become more human because they are matters of choice, not chance.[9]

Several features of Fletcher's argument require careful scrutiny. Note first that he regards the generation of human life as an act of reproduction: babies are entities that we "make." They are, as it were, products of our artistic creativity, and since these "products" can be more deliberately "designed" and planned by the use of various techniques of artful childmaking than they can be by the "random" selection of what Fletcher elsewhere terms "reproductive roulette,"[10] it follows that it is more human to "make" them in a controlled and designed way than to "make" them haphazardly. The notion that a child is a product is one to which we shall return.

Note secondly Fletcher's notion of human intelligence. He evidently considers human intelligence as primarily a "technical reason," that is, the ability to plan and organize and arrange means efficiently to reach predetermined ends.[11] This indeed is one aspect of human intelligence; it is what enables us to make efficient use of our time, to "control" nature and to create the world of human art and culture. Yet our existence as intelligent creatures is by no means exhausted by this function of our minds. Fletcher here seems to equate human intelligence with but one of its functions, namely its artistic, creative function, and to ignore other crucially significant intellectual operations, in particular its contemplative operation of discovering the truth about reality and its moral or ethical operation of putting order into our lives by directing choice according to objective norms of morality.[12] It is surely possible that there are some things that we can "make" (e.g., thermonuclear bombs whose only possible purpose is to destroy entire peoples) that we will come to know we ought not to make because the choice to do so is contrary to normative principles of human action.[13] The issue before us is whether we ought to choose to "make" babies by laboratory techniques. Here I suggest that Fletcher and those who accept his argument simply fail to face this issue and beg the question by focussing onesidedly upon one aspect of human intelligence.

Next note Fletcher's contention—one that is, I fear, shared by many in our culture today—that there is nothing morally problematic about our ability to sever completely the bonds linking the untive, amative, or "love-making" (I would prefer to say "love-giving") meaning of our genital sexuality and its procreative or, as Fletcher describes it, its "reproductive" or "baby-making" aspect. Here Fletcher expresses agreement with all who would agree with Ashley Montagu in saying that "it is necessary to be unequivocally clear concerning the distinction between *sexual* behavior and *reproductive* behavior."[14] They are two radically different sorts of human activity, governed by radically different sorts of rules. Since in vitro fertilization and other modes of artful childmaking require the intentional choice to sever the connection between the unitive or amative and the propagative meaning of a human person's genital sexuality, this is obviously a central issue, and to it I shall return.

In his comments on the position taken by Fletcher and others of similar mind, McCormick observed that it rests on three assumptions: (1) "a consequentialistic or teleological[15] normative position," according to which an act or practice is right and good "if, on balance, it does more good than harm and helps to minimize human suffering;" (2) a sharp distinction (one I have already noted) "between sexual love and the generation of human life;" and (3) a conception of parenthood "as a relationship essentially and principally defined by acts of nurturing, not by acts of begetting."[16]

McCormick's comments on the position taken by Fletcher are important for several reasons. First, they call to our attention two features in this position–its consequentialistic moral methodology and its understanding of parenthood–that were not explicitly brought out in the passage from Fletcher previously considered. And the features McCormick notes are quite central to the broad justification that this position provides not only for in vitro fertilization by married couples to alleviate infertility but also for all sorts of reproductive interventions.

Second, McCormick's comments will help us understand the presuppositions behind another position, one more cautious and nuanced than that advocated by Fletcher and his colleagues, that is used to justify the practice of in vitro fertilization when this is strictly limited to helping *married couples* otherwise childless have a child of their own. I shall now turn to consider this position.

Its general contours are well described by McCormick. Thus it will be useful, to begin discussion of it, to see how McCormick describes its underlying assumptions. McCormick writes as follows concerning those who adopt this more cautious justification of in vitro fertilization for married couples:

> First, they are not pure teleologists [by this he means consequentialistic teleologists, cf. note 15] in their moral thinking–that is, they argue that factors other than consequences need to be taken into account in offering a valid ethical evaluation of any human act, although many such writers do believe that a proportionately good enough end can justify the deliberate, direct intent to effect some kinds of disvalues and evils. Second, they maintain that a meaningful and reciprocal relationship between sexual love and the generation of human life exists and that it is no mere evolutionary accident that human life comes into existence through an act that is also capable of expressing love be-

> tween a man and a woman. Third, while recognizing that acts of nurturing life are distinct from acts of generating life and that acts of nurturing are included within the meaning of parenthood, they also affirm that acts of generating life are parental in nature and carry with them responsibilities for nurturing the life procreated.[17]

I believe that McCormick has well described the general presuppositions shared by several authors, including such Roman Catholic theologians as Johannes Gründel, Charles E. Curran, and McCormick himself,[18] who have come to the conclusion that in vitro fertilization, when restricted to helping alleviate the problems of *married persons* and utilizing gametic material provided by the spouses, *can be* a morally good choice provided other conditions are met. These writers also, it can be noted incidentally, hold that husband artificial insemination can also be morally justifiable. First I wish to call attention to some of the other conditions that must be met, in the judgment of these writers, for this practice to be morally acceptable. I shall then comment briefly on their assumptions.

One of the most important other conditions that must be met, according to these writers, in order to justify resorting to in vitro fertilization, is that serious harm to the child-to-be from the procedure itself must be reasonably excluded. In short, these writers recognize that in vitro fertilization constitutes a medical experimentation upon a human subject—in this case the child-to-be—and that it would be morally wrong to expose this subject to serious and unknown risks in order to satisfy the desires of other human subjects, e.g., their parents. Here they are thinking of the very serious objection to in vitro fertilization raised initially by Paul Ramsey and Leon Kass.[19] Thus to understand the concern of these writers it is important to grasp the problem raised by Ramsey and Kass. I shall present the problem in the form given to it by Ramsey. To understand his argument it is first necessary to be clear about a crucial matter. The human subject with whose well-being Ramsey is concerned, in posing his objection to in vitro fertilization, is the child-to-be in the sense of the child who will eventually be born as a result of the procedure. Thus in presenting his problem Ramsey prescinds from the question of the moral status of the living entity existing here and now in the laboratory petri dish after fertilization or of the developing unborn entity in utero after implantation. The subject upon whom Ramsey claims that an unethical experimentation is being done is thus not the living being existing in the laboratory after fertilization (and that may be "discarded" prior to implantation should any discernible abnormality develop) nor is it the living being in utero that may be aborted should amniocentesis (performed, it should be noted, late in pregnancy) disclose that it may possibly be afflicted with a serious malady. Rather the subject of the unethical experimentation in Ramsey's argument is the child-to-be, the child who is *not yet* in being after fertilization and during pregnancy but who will be in being after birth.

Ramsey argued that in vitro fertilization is an unethical experimentation on *this* subject "*unless* the *possibility* of irreparable damage to this child-to-be can be definitively excluded." He then continued by saying, "this condition cannot be met, at least not by the first 'successful cases.' "[20] By this he meant that this condition has not even now, after the birth of Louise Brown and a few other children, apparently normal, as a result of in vitro fertilization, been met because we do not know *yet* whether some harm later to be suffered may have been induced by the procedure itself. Briefly, Ramsey claimed that researchers simply cannot "*exclude* the possibility that they will do irreparable damage to the child to be."[21] They cannot know, *nor can they ever come to know,* what possible harm they are doing to this possible future child *without being willing to inflict such damage in order to find out.*[22] And this, Ramsey argued, is an irresponsible and unwarranted injustice to this child to be.

Those defending the moral rightness of in vitro fertilization by married couples recognize the serious problem that Ramsey raised. They nonetheless claim that his position is too stringent. Were it true, they argue, then it would even be immoral for married couples to choose to have children through normal marital relations, inasmuch as they cannot absolutely exclude the possibility that the child they engender may be irrevocably and irreparably harmed in its coming-to-be because of unknown recessive genetic defects or mutations.[23] They therefore hold that the moral issue raised by Ramsey can be better expressed in normative terms if we stipulate that one necessary conditon that must be met prior to resorting to in vitro fertilization is the reasonable expectation that the risks to which the child-to-be will be subjected will be less than or equivalent to those that might reasonably be expected in normal generation through marital coition.[24] Whether or not this prior conditon can be met is a matter that can only be settled by scientific data, and on this, at present, authorities are divided.[25]

Another condition that must be met, according to these authors, if in vitro fertilization is to be rightly used, is an unwillingness to abort a child conceived through this process and implanted in its mother's womb, should some abnormality develop. At least this is a condition that several of the authors adopting this position require.[26] Those who accept this position are likewise concerned about the problem of "discarding" fertilized ova prior to implantation. As originally practiced by Steptoe and Edwards, in vitro fertilization usually required the fertilization of several ova removed from the mother (who had been given onovulatory drugs) by her husband's sperm, the monitoring of their development in the petri dish, and the implantation within the mother's womb of that developing life judged most promising to continue development in utero and the "discarding" of those not chosen for implantation. Although most of the writers accepting the view now under consideration are of the mind that individual personal life is not present prior to implantation and that therefore the developing human lives in petri dishes prior to implantation are not personal subjects with a right to life in a strong sense, they are nonetheless very much concerned about the problem of "wastage" and of "discarded" zygotes. Thus many of them add as a further condition for the morally legitimate use of in vitro fertilization by married couples the stipulation that only one ovum from the mother be fertilized by her husband's sperm and that there be the intention to implant the resultant human life within her womb.[27]

I will forego commentary on the issues raised by these conditions so that attention can focus on the basic underlying assumptions of the authors who propose that in vitro fertilization, once these conditions are fulfilled, may be rightfully chosen by married couples as a way of fulfilling their desire for a child of their own so long as the wife's ovum is fertilized by her husband's sperm.

The third assumption of these authors that McCormick notes, namely that acts of generating life are parental and carry with them the responsibility to nurture the life generated, poses no problems in my opinion. Here these authors are quite correct. They simply remind us of the responsibilities that we freely take upon ourselves in freely choosing to exercise our procreative sexuality. Their further insistence that parenting is not exhausted by generating activities but requires nurturing activities is also eminently sound. Unlike Fletcher and his colleagues they refuse to see a dichotomy between generating and nurturing activities; they refuse to reduce the former to merely biological and nonparental behavior and to erect the latter alone to the level of parental behavior. So far, so good. But what can be said about their other two assumptions?

Note that these authors, in the first assumption listed by McCormick, reject the kind of consequentialistic thinking employed by Fletcher. Nonetheless, as McCormick himself observed, many of them "do believe that a proportionately good enough end can justify the deliberate, direct intent to effect some kinds of disvalues and evils." I submit that these authors, while eschewing the simplistic consequentialism of Fletcher and his associates, are nonetheless consequentialistic teleologists in their normative ethical theory inasmuch as they justify "exceptions" to the moral norms they develop (whether on consequentialistic or nonconsequentialistic grounds) on the basis of a consequentialistic criterion, that namely of the alleged "greater good." With McCormick they contend that it is morally right to choose to do a (premoral) evil for the sake of some greater (premoral) good to come. In this instance, they are willing to choose to sever the bond linking the intimate genital expression of marital love to the generation of human life—and they obviously believe that this bond is something very good so that the choice to sever it is indeed the choice to do an evil or disvalue—because the choice to do *this* evil is ordered to the accomplishing of something they regard as an even greater good, namely the generation of a child ardently desired by the couple. These authors thus subscribe to the consequentialistic proposition that *it is morally right to choose to do (premoral) evil for the sake of a proportionately greater (premoral) good.*

To enter here into an extensive discussion of normative ethical theory and to show in detail why this presupposition of the authors under consideration is erroneous would take us too far afield. Still I can briefly pose the most devastating objection to this consequentialistic position. This normative position assumes that the various real goods of human existence—the "premoral" goods in question—can in some way be measured or weighed against each other prior to choice so that one can judge in an unambiguous and unequivocal way that some of these goods are measurably greater than others and that goods of lesser value can then be destroyed or cast aside or impeded if their continued flourishing inhibits participation in the "higher" or "greater" goods of human existence. But this assumption is erroneous and is so because the goods in question are simply incalculable and incommensurable. The effort to weigh or measure them off against another or in terms of some common denominator is akin to the effort to compare the number 784 with the length of a rainbow. An abundant literature exists on this subject.[28] Indeed, so fruitless have been the efforts of proportionalistic consequentialists to show that the commensuration they require is possible that one of their leading spokesmen, McCormick, has been compelled to admit that the goods are indeed incommensurable but to follow this admission with the assertion that nonetheless we must, "in fear and trembling," commensurate them by waging prudent bets.[29] What this shows us, I submit, is that the consequentialistic proportionalist is ultimately forced to admit that the commensuration he requires is in fact impossible and then to attempt to settle the matter by arbitrarily declaring that his preferences for certain goods-those upon which he places his bets, i.e., those that he *chooses* to prefer to others–shows that these goods are greater than the ones he chooses to get rid of because they inhibit his participation in the ones he prefers. Thus rather than providing us with a principle whereby we can *judge* what ought to be done *prior* to choice, the proportionalist simply settles the matter *by making a choice* and then attempts to justify the choice.

A final assumption of these authors is that the procreative and unitive meanings of our genital sexuality go together and are meant to go together. As McCormick put it, "they maintain that a meaningful and reciprocal relationship between sexual love and the generation of human life exists and that it is no mere evolutionary accident that human life comes into existence through an act that is also capable of expressing love between a man and a woman[I think it would have been better put had McCormick written, 'between a husband and his wife.' "] They thus wish to keep the generation of human life within the marital covenant and to exclude the use of in vitro fertilization by nonmarried persons or linking it to such features as donor sperm and/or ova, surrogate or host mothers, etc. They see marriage, marital coition, and the generation of human life as inherently interrelated, and they regard this inherent interrelationship as something of great human value, one that must be respected.

Nonetheless, they conclude that the choice by married couples to resort to the laboratory generation of human life—specifically of a child they ardently wish to have—may be justified (under the conditions already noted) even though this choice does entail the severing of the bond uniting the unitive or love-giving and the procreative or life-giving meanings of genital sexuality. They hold, in other words, that it is morally permissible to choose to generate human life by acts that are not those of marital coition but rather those of persons skilled in the employment of contemporary biological knowledge and technology. For them the laboratory generation of human life, even though it is itself an act of generating that life outside of the marital act and of necessity entails the choice to separate the life-giving aspect of genital sexuality from its love-giving aspect, is morally good provided that the married couple provide the gametic cells to be used in the fertilization, that the mother nurture the life thus generated, and that the couple then nurture the child eventually born.

This more limited defense of in vitro fertilization, accepted by several contemporary authors, including a number of Roman Catholic theologians, thus recognizes that the generation of human life is inherently and intimately linked to marriage and that human life ought to be generated in the marital act, the act that communicates both love and life. But they believe that we can, under very limited conditions and after satisfying stringent requirements, rightly choose to generate human life outside of the marital act through the laboratory process of in vitro fertilization. As one of their exponents, McCormick, has put it, "it seems very difficult to reject *in vitro* fertilization with embryo transfer [to help a married couple otherwise childless achieve an ardently desired pregnancy] on the sole ground of artificiality or the separation of the unitive and the procreative . . . unless one accepts this physical inseparability as an inviolable norm."[30]

Obviously these authors' acceptance of the proportionalist criterion for justifying exceptions to moral norms plays a major role in their argument. They recognize as a genuine moral norm that human life ought to be given in and through the marital act and they acknowledge that the choice to generate a human outside of this act includes a choice to do (premoral) evil, but they contend that the deliberate choice to do this evil is justified by the even greater (premoral) good that it will bring about. Thus their position can and ought to be challenged on the grounds that it rests upon the prior acceptance of a normative moral norm (the proportionalist criterion). Nonetheless, in the following section of this essay I will concentrate attention not so much on the moral methodology employed as on the profound human significance of the bond linking marriage, the marital act, and the generation of human life. In this way I hope to show that the basic objection to the laboratory generation of human life is *not,* as McCormick claims, the *physical inseparability*[31] of the unitive and procreative meanings of the marital act but rather the deliberate choice to generate human life nonmaritally.

3. *The Basic Reason Why It Is Morally Wrong to Choose to Generate Human Life in the Laboratory*

Perhaps a good way to begin is to review briefly pertinent Church teaching on the subject. In 1949 Pope Pius XII, in rejecting artificial insemination by a husband, had this to say:

> We must never forget this: It is only the procreation of a new life *according to the will and plan of the Creator* which brings with it—to an astonishing degree of perfection—the realization of the desired ends. This is, at the same time, in harmony with the dignity of the marriage partners, with their bodily and spiritual natures, and with the normal and happy development of the child.[32]

Evidently Pius XII was of the mind that God wills that human life be begotton *only* in the marital act and that the choice to generate it outside of the marital act is a choice that goes against God's will. In 1951 he returned to the subject, now asserting this:

> To reduce the cohabitation of married persons and the conjugal act to a mere organic function for the transmission of the germs of life would be to convert the domestic hearth, sanctuary of the family, into nothing more than a biological laboratory . . . The conjugal act in its natural structure is a personal action, a simultaneous natural self-giving which, in the words of Holy Scripture, effects the union "in one flesh." This is more than the mere union of two germs, which can be brought about artificially—i.e., without the natural action of the spouses. The conjugal act as it is planned and willed by nature implies a personal cooperation, the right to which parties have mutually conferred on each other in contracting marriage.[33]

Here Pius XII indicates that the reason why human life ought to be given *only* in and through the act of intimate conjugal love and *ought not* to be generated in the laboraory is that only in this way—one planned and willed by nature and by God—is it truly a personal act of the married couple, one to which they and they alone have a right. The assumption is that human life ought only to be generated in a personal act of the married couple.

Although later pontiffs have not directly addressed the issue of the laboratory generation of human life, their teaching on marriage and its relationship to the giving of human life clearly shows that they are of the same mind as Pius XII. Thus Pope Paul VI insisted that the Church has always taught as inviolable

> the inseparable connection, willed by God and unable to be broken by man on his own initiative, between the two meanings of the conjugal act: the unitive meaning and the procreative meaning. Indeed, by its intimate structure the conjugal act, while most closely uniting husband and wife, capacitates them for the generation of new lives, according to laws inscribed in the very being of man and of woman. By safeguarding both these essential aspects, the unitive and the procreative, the conjugal act preserves in its fullness the sense of true mutual love and its ordination towards man's most high calling to parenthood.[34]

It is instructive, I believe, to note that Pope Paul here insists that the conjugal act—the act in which husband and wife share their own persons and their powers of genital sexuality with its love-giving and life-giving dimensions—*capacitates* the spouses to generate new human life. In speaking of the inviolable bond between the unitive and procreative meanings of the marital act, Paul VI was, of course, primarily intending to show why the choice to contracept is immoral; still his teaching on the inviolable bond between these two meanings of the conjugal act is obviously relevant to the question concerning the morality of the choice to sever this bond so that one can generate life in an act that is not also one in which the spouses share their persons in an intimacy of love.

Finally, Pope John Paul II, in his stirring homily to the great crowd assembled for Mass on the Capitol Mall of Washington D.C. on October 7, 1979, insisted that human life is precious not only because it is a gift from a loving God but also because "it is the expression and the fruit of love." Continuing, he said, "This is why life should spring up within the setting of marriage."[35] Clearly he indicates here that the generation of human life ought only to be brought about within the covenant of marriage.

The Roman Catholic authors who justify in vitro fertilization for married couples under very stringent conditions are, of course, aware of these papal teachings. Still they believe that the insistence in these teachings that there is an inviolable bond between the unitive and the procreative meanings of the conjugal act cannot be sustained. McCormick suggests that the papal objection to the sundering of this bond, even when the choice to do is made to help a married couple otherwise childless to have a child of their own, rests upon the belief that the choice to sunder the bond is dehumanizing and hence immoral. This belief, he suggests, is a kind of intuition. The problem with this, he then notes, is that "intuitions notoriously differ" and that other reasonable persons entertain different intuitions about the matter.[36] He likewise suggests, as I have already noted, that the papal teaching seems to erect the *physical inseparability* of the procreative and the unitive meanings of the conjugal act into a moral norm.

I believe that these papal teachings are true and that they are an endeavor, on the part of the Church expressing its mind through their teachings, to remind some critically important truths about the meaning of human existence. I believe that these teachings can be shown to be true, and I propose to show them to be true by offering the following argument. I will first put it in the form of a syllogism and then seek to establish the truth of the major and minor premises. The argument can be formulated as follows:

> Any act of generating human life that is nonmarital is irresponsible and violates the reverence due to human life in its generation.
>
> But in vitro fertilization and other forms of the laboratory generation of human life, including artificial insemination whether by vendor or husband, are nonmarital.
>
> Therefore these modes of generating human life are irresponsible and violate the reverence due to human life in its generation.

In my opinion the minor premise does not require extensive discussion. Artificial insemination by a vendor is evidently nonmarital, and the same is obviously true of in vitro fertilization involving the use of ova and/or sperm from persons who are not married to each other. Moreover even artificial insemination by a husband and in vitro fertilization in which an ovum taken from the wife is fertilized by sperm provided by her husband are also nonmarital in nature, even though married persons or spouses have collaborated in the procedure. Such procedures are nonmarital because they are *in principle* procedures that may be effected by persons who are not spouses; in addition and more significantly, the spousal character of the man and woman participating in the procedures is not intrinsic to the procedures even though they may happen to be husband and wife. What makes husband and wife capable of participating in such activities is not their spousal union but the simple fact that they are beings who produce gametic cells, ova in the case of the woman and sperm in the case of the man.

The major premise is the one that in my judgment needs argument for its truth to become manifest. To show why it is true I think it is necessary first to reflect on the meaning of marriage, marital love, and the marital act and then to show why the choice to engender human life nonmaritally is so destructive of goods crucial to human existence.

Marriage does not derive from faith in Jesus and membership in His body, the Church. Nonetheless the human reality of marriage, which is in truth a loving gift of God to the human race,[37] is a reality inherently capable of being integrated into God's covenant of love and grace. In and through Christ it has indeed been so integrated for those who experience this reality "in the Lord," that is, as living members of His spouse the Church.[38] Moreover even the marriages of men and women who have not yet heard the gospel message "are included in a certain inchoative way in the marital love which unites Christ with his church."[39]

The beautiful reality of marriage comes into being through an act "of irrevocable personal consent . . . whereby the spouses mutually bestow and accept each other."[40] This act, which *alone* can bring marriage into being,[41] is comparable to that irrevocable act whereby God has freely chosen us as the beings with whom and for whom He wills to share His life and love and to that irrevocable act whereby His only-begotten Son, become one with us in His humanity, has freely chosen to become indissolubly one with His bride, the Church. In and through this act a man and a woman give to themselves a new identity: he becomes *her* husband and she becomes *his* wife and together they become *spouses*. This act of mutual bestowal establishes the man and the woman as uniquely irreplaceable and non-substitutable spouses.[42] In and through this act that brings marriage into being the man and the woman surrender to one another their person, including their sexuality with its procreative and unitive aspects. Moreover, in making themselves to be husband and wife a man and a woman promise conjugal or marital love to one another: in virtue of this act and of the marriage that it brings into being they have henceforward the right, the freedom, and the obligation to love each other with conjugal love.[43] In addition, "marriage and marital love are ordered to the procreation and education of the offspring and it is in them that marriage finds it crowning glory."[44]

Marital or spousal love is a unique form of human love, and what makes it to be unique is the fact that it is an exclusive kind of love. Yet its exclusive character needs to be rightly understood. Husband and wife, through conjugal love, are not locked in an *égoisme à deux,* one cutting them off from other persons or excluding love of other persons.[45] Quite to the contrary, they are enabled, precisely by virtue of their marriage and their exclusive spousal love, one "merging the human with the divine,"[46] to realize "the goodness and loveableness of all people, in fact of all living things."[47] Nor is conjugal love exclusive in the sense that husband and wife are the "property" of each other. Such possessive language is totally foreign to and destructive of marriage and marital love.[48] Rather conjugal love is exclusive in that it is rooted in the irrevocable choice, by the spouses, of each other as *the* one with whom and for whom each will henceforth share a common life in marriage, a life too in which they are dynamically inclined to share their person intimately with one another in the marital act and in that act to give life and love to new human persons.[49]

The exclusive character of marital love, the character that specifies it and distinguishes it from every other form of human friendship love can perhaps be best understood by reflecting on the significance of the act of which spouses, and spouses alone, are capable, namely the marital or conjugal act. Although the spouses may freely choose never to engage in this act,[50] and although this act is not necessarily the *greatest* expression of conjugal love,[51] it is certainly true that marriage is ordered to this act in a dynamic way[52] and that it is the act in which exclusive marital love is "uniquely expressed and perfected."[53]

The marital act is the act of marital coition. This act

exhibits, symbolizes, manifests the exclusive nature of marital love, and it does so because it is both a communion in being (conjugal love as unitive) and is the sort or kind of act in and through which the spouses are "open to the transmission of life,"[54] in which, as Pope John Paul II has put it, they submit their being to the blessing of fertility[55] (conjugal love as procreative).

The marital act is unitive, i.e., a communion in being or an intimate, exclusive sharing of personal life because through it and in it husband and wife come to know one another in a unique way, revealing themselves to one another. In and through it they become one flesh, that is, humanly and personally one, renewing the covenant they have made with each other in the act that made them to be spouses.[56] Moreover, in this act husband and wife exhibit their sexual complementarity as male and female; for this act is possible only because the male, who has a penis, is personally able to enter into the person of the female, and she is uniquely capable of receiving personally into her body, her person, the male; and her act of receiving in a giving sort of way is just as central to the meaning of this act as is the male's act of giving his person to her in a receiving sort of way.[57] The husband cannot, in this act, give himself to his wife (i.e., exercise the unitive power of his sexuality), unless she gives herself to him by receiving him, nor can the wife receive him in this self-giving way by the exercise of the unitive power of her sexuality unless he gives himself to her by letting himself be received by her.

The marital act is procreative insofar as it is the kind or sort of act—and the kind or sort of act *alone*—that makes it possible for husband and wife to exercise *maritally* their beautiful personal and sexual powers of procreation, of giving life to a new human person. It is, in short, the sort or kind of act that is "open to the transmission of life" in a marital, procreative way.

And finally, this act is *marital* because it is an act that *only* spouses can do. Unmarried persons may be able to engage in sexual coition, but since they have not made themselves to be non-substitutable and irreplaceable spouses through the act that brings marriage into being, such acts are in no way the manifestation of an exclusive sort of love.[58] Unmarried persons may also be able to generate life through sexual coition, but such acts of generating human life are by no means acts of procreative love. Moreover, this act is *marital* not only because married persons *alone* can do it, but also because it is the *only* sort or kind that married persons can do that other persons cannot do. In addition, if married persons engage in genital sex and in so doing choose either to repudiate its exclusively unitive nature by having disregard for or even contempt for the feelings of each other or to repudiate its openness to the transmission of life, they are not choosing to engage in the marital act but are rather making the act they choose to engage in something other than the marital act.[59]

In the light of these reflections on marriage, marital love, and the marital act, I believe that we can see why the deliberate choice to generate human life nonmaritally is irresponsible. It is irresponsible, first of all, because it is in essence a choice that attacks the great good of marriage itself. Marriage, exclusive marital love, and the procreation of new human life through the marital act are goods that go together. To attack one of these goods is to attack and do violence to the others. Our age sufficiently bears witness to the destruction done to the great human reality of marriage by denying the exclusive yet nonpossessive character of marital love, for we now have many who seriously propose mate-swapping and "creative" adultery,[60] and by denying the goodness of spousal procreativity, for many not only endorse contraceptive practices but claim that many married persons do not have a right to procreate.[61] To choose to sever the bond joining marriage, the marital act, and the generation of human life is further to threaten the good of marriage itself and is thus irresponsible. Yet this is precisely what is done when one adopts by choice the proposal to generate human life in acts that are by their very nature nonmarital.

There is, in addition, a further matter that must be taken

into account in thinking about the choice to separate the generation of human life from the procreative marital act. This is the truth that a human life, the life of a being that is the bearer of inviolable and inalienable rights, is not to be considered as a product inferior in nature and subordinate in value to its producers. Rather a human life is concretely an irreplaceable being of moral worth, a person. For a Christian, moreover, a human life is in truth a living word of God, a created word vicariously imaging God Himself. The Christian remembers, too, that God's Uncreated Word became, for love of us, a created word. And the Uncreated Word who became and is still a created word, a fellow member of our species, is a Word that is, as we affirm in the Creed, "begotten, not made." Thus we, the created words of God, brothers and sisters of the eternally begotten Word of the Father, are to be begotten, not made. Human life, therefore, is meant to be begotten in and through the marital act, which is as it were a word spoken by husband and wife in which they affirm that they are open both to sharing life and love with each other and to sharing life and love with a new human life, a being who, like them, is irreplaceable and precious. It is therefore irresponsible to choose to produce this life through the nonmarital act of fertilizing ova with sperm. Such an act may "make" a baby, and the baby[62] made by such an act is indeed a precious and irreplaceable human life worthy of the same respect and reverence due to all other human lives; yet such an act is not one of begetting human life in a procreative way.

To sum up, the choice to generate human life in the laboratory, insofar as it is a choice to reproduce human life nonmaritally, is irresponsible because it is a choice that threatens the good of marriage itself and by so doing endangers human life in its generation; it is likewise a choice that violates the reverence due to human life in its generation insofar as it transforms the act of generating human life from one of procreative marital love to one of artistic production, thereby treating human life not as a good of incomparable and priceless value but rather as a product subordinate to its producers.

Some may perhaps think that the position taken here is heartless and unconcerned with the anguish experienced by married couples who ardently desire a child of their own and must suffer disappointment because of a pathological condition. I do not believe that it is. Their desire for a child of their own is a truly noble and generous one. But the moral question centers not on this desire but on the human deeds freely chosen in order to satisfy it. An authentically human ethics is one that is as concerned with means as it is with ends, for we can choose to do some dreadful deeds with the best of intentions and with the noblest of ends in view.

Moreover, for married couples with the dilemma of those who cannot have a child because of blocked fallopian tubes there are alternative possibilities. Surgical reconstruction of the fallopian tubes is currently possible in approximately thirty percent of cases—a far higher success rate than efforts to "produce" children through in vitro fertilization, and such reconstruction is truly therapeutic of a human pathology, whereas in vitro fertilization leaves the pathology untouched and simply helps fulfill desires. Moreover, it has been suggested that it may be possible to remove the ovum from the ovaries, implant it in the fallopian tube below the point where the tube is blocked, and then have husband and wife unite in the act of marital love.[63] This procedure, should it prove workable, is in my judgment morally permissible, and offers great hope for those married couples for whom the laboratory generation of human life is now proposed.[64]

In concluding, I wish simply to suggest that the crucial issue posed by the laboratory generation of human life is the bond uniting marriage, the marital act, and the begetting of human life. I hold that human life, the life that the Word eternally begotten by the Father united to His divinity, is a life meant to be begotten, not made. It is begotten in and through the marital act; it is made in the laboratory.

NOTES

1. Pope Paul VI, *Humanae Vitae*, n. 12.
2. James Watson, "Moving Toward the Clonal Man: Is This What We Want?" *The Atlantic* (May, 1971) 50-53.
3. I use the term "vendor" advisedly. George J. Annas, a lawyer, has pointed out that the term "donor" is a misnomer and that those males who provide artificial insemination in women whom they do not even know are more truthfully described as "sperm vendors." Annas wrote: "It is a contract in which the vendor is agreeing to do certain things for pay . . . The continued use of the term "donor" gives the impression that the sperm vendor is doing some service for the good of humanity." "Artificial Insemination: Beyond the Best Interests of the Donor," *Hastings Center Report* 9.4 (August, 1979) 14-15, 43.
4. Richard A. McCormick, S.J., *How Brave a New World: Dilemmas in Bioethics* (Garden City, N.Y.: Doubleday, 1981), pp. 308-312.
5. *Ibid.*, pp. 309-311.
6. One issue, largely ignored in considering amniocentesis followed by abortion in the event that a "defective" fetus is discovered, is the problem of falsely identifying as actually afflicted by a genetic malady a fetus that is not. For a superb study of this matter see Paul Ramsey, "Screening: An Ethicist's View," in *Ethical Issues in Human Genetics*, ed. Bruce Hilton et al. (New York: Plenum Press, 1973), pp. 150-155.
7. On the serious legal and social issues that this "solution" raises see Annas, "Artificial Insemination."
8. Joseph F. Fletcher, "Ethical Aspects of Genetic Controls: Designed Genetic Changes in Man," *New England Journal of Medicine* 285 (1971) 776-783; Robert Francoeur, *Utopian Motherhood: New Trends in Human Reproduction* (Garden City, N.Y.: Doubleday, 1970); Michael Hamilton, "New Life for Old: Genetic Decision," *Christian Century* 86 (1969) 743.
9. Fletcher, "Ethical Aspects of Genetic Controls," 781-782.
10. This is the subtitle that Fletcher gave to his book, *The Ethics of Genetic Control: Ending Reproductive Roulette* (Garden City, N.Y.: Doubleday Anchor, 1974).
11. On this see Nicholas Crotty, "The Technological Imperative: Reflection on Reflections," *Theological Studies* 33.3 (September, 1972) 441-447.
12. On this subject it is instructive to read Thomas Aquinas, *In Decem Libros Ethicorum Aristotelis Expositio* (Rome: Marietti, 1955), Liber I, lectio 1, n. 2.
13. I am not claiming that making a thermonuclear bomb is in and of itself immoral, but making such bombs for the precise purpose of obliterating populations is and making bombs that could only be used for this purpose is immoral.
14. Ashley Montagu, *Sex, Man and Culture* (New York: Putnam, 1969), pp. 13-14. For a critique of this "separatist" view of human sexuality see my *Sex, Marriage, and Chastity: Reflections of a Catholic Layman, Spouse, and Parent* (Chicago: Franciscan Herald Press, 1981), ch. 1.

15. McCormick confuses matters, I believe, by using "consequentialistic" and "teleological" as synonyms. A teleological ethical theory, as opposed to a formalistic, duty oriented deontological theory, need not be consequentialistic. For a good presentation of this matter see Germain G. Grisez and Joseph M. Boyle, Jr., *Life and Death With Liberty and Justice: A Contribution to the Euthanasia Debate* (Notre Dame, Ind.: University of Notre Dame Press, 1978), pp. 345-361. See also Frederick S. Carney, "On McCormick and Teleological Morality," *Journal of Religious Ethics* 6 (Spring, 1978) 81-107.
16. McCormick, *How Brave a New World?*, p. 311.
17. *Ibid*, p. 312.
18. Johannes Gründel, "Zeugung in der Retorte-unsittlich?" *Stimmen der Zeit* 103 (1978) 675-682; Charles E. Curran, *Politics, Medicine, and Christian Ethics* (Philadelphia: Fortress, 1973), pp. 200-219; McCormick, *How Brave a New World?*, pp. 306-325.
19. Leon Kass, "Making Babies: The New Biology and the 'Old' Morality," *The Public Interest* 26 (Winter, 1972) 28-56; Kass, "Babies by Means of *In Vitro* Fertilization: Unethical Experiments on the Unborn?" *New England Journal of Medicine* 285 (1971) 1174-1179; Paul Ramsey, "Shall We 'Reproduce'? I. The Medical Ethics of *In Vitro* Fertilization," *Journal of the American Medical Association* 220 (1972) 1346-1350; Ramsey, "Shall We 'Reproduce'? II. Rejoinders and Future Forecast," *Journal of the American Medical Association* 220 (1972) 1480-1485. Kass later returned to this subject in his 'Making Babies' Revisited," *The Public Interest* 54 (Winter, 1979) 32-59. In his more recent article Kass, while still arguing against in vitro fertilization, suggests that the risk of harm need not be positively excluded. It is sufficient if it is equivalent to or less than the risks to the child from normal procreation.
20. Ramsey, "Shall We 'Reproduce'? I.," 1347.
21. *Ibid.*
22. *Ibid.*
23. See, for instance, Curran, *Politics, Medicine, and Christian Ethics*, p. 212.
24. McCormick, *How Brave a New World?*, p. 331.
25. For an extensive survey of the pertinent literature on this see LeRoy Walters, "Human In Vitro Fertilization: A Review of the Literature," *Hastings Center Report* 9.4 (August, 1979) 23-43, especially p. 27 for the scientific literature.
26. For instance, McCormick, *How Brave a New World?*, p. 332.
27. *Ibid.*
28. The best essay on this subject is Germain G. Grisez, "Against Consequentialism," *American Journal of Jurisprudence* 23 (1978) 21-72. The argument given there is well summarized by Grisez and Joseph M. Boyle, *Life and Death With Liberty and Justice*, pp. 346-358. Other important literature showing the difficulties with consequentialism and proportionalism includes: Carney, "On McCormick and Teleological Morality;" Ramsey, "Incommensurability and Indeterminancy in Moral Choice," in *Doing Evil to Achieve Good: Moral Choice in Conflict Situations*, ed. Richard A. McCormick, S.J. and Paul Ramsey (Chicago: Loyola University

Press, 1978), pp. 69-144; John F. Connery, "Catholic Ethics: Has the Norm for Rule-Making Changed?," *Theological Studies* 42.2 (June, 1981) 232-250; William E. May, *Becoming Human: an Invitation to Christian Ethics* (Dayton: Pflaum, 1974), ch. 4. The argument for consequentialism/proportionalism is found in the following: Richard A. McCormick, S.J., *Ambiguity in Moral Choice* (Milwaukee: Department of Theology Marquette University, 1973), reprinted in *Doing Evil to Achieve Good,* pp. 7-53; McCormick, "A Commentary on the Commentaries," in *Doing Evil to Achieve Good,* pp. 193-267; the essays by Bruno Schüller, Josef Fuchs, Peter Knauer, Franz Scholz, Louis Janssens, McCormick, Curran and others in *Readings in Moral Theology. I. Moral Norms and the Catholic Tradition* (New York: Paulist Press, 1979; this volume also includes essays by Paul Quay, S.J. and John Connery, S.J. in opposition to the consequentialistic position). See also the essays by Richard Roach, William E. May, John Finnis, and Germain G. Grisez in *Principles of Catholic Moral Life,* ed. William E. May (Chicago: Franciscan Herald Press, 1981).

29. McCormick, "Commentary on the Commentaries," pp. 227-230.
30. McCormick, *How Brave a New World?,* pp. 328-329.
31. This raises the issue of physicalism, a charge frequently made by those theologians who opposed the teaching on contraception given in *Humanae Vitae*. McCormick here echoes this charge with respect to the teaching on in vitro fertilization. The claim of physicalism is pressed by many of the contributors (e.g. Daniel C. Maguire, Charles E. Curran, and Bernard Häring) to *Contraception: Authority and Dissent,* ed. Charles E. Curran (New York: Herder and Herder, 1969). The charge has been critically assessed and refuted by many writers. See, for instance, William E. May, *Sex, Love, and Procreation* (Chicago: Franciscan Herald Press Synthesis Series, 1976); Germain G. Grisez, "Dualism and the New Morality," *Atti del Congresso Internazionale (Roma-Napoli-17/24 Aprile 1974) Tommaso d'Aquino nel suo Settimo Centenario,* vol. 5, *L'Agire Morale* (Napoli: Edizioni Domenicane Italiane, 1977), pp. 323-330.
32. Pope Pius XII, "To Catholic Doctors: An Address by His Holiness to the Fourth International Convention of Catholic Doctors, Castelgondolfo, Italy, September 29, 1949," *Catholic Mind* 48 (1950) 250-253.
33. Pope Pius XII, "Apostolate of the Midwives: An Address by His Holiness to the Italian Catholic Union of Midwives, October 29, 1951," *Catholic Mind* 50 (1952) 61.
34. Pope Paul VI, *Humanae Vitae,* n. 12.
35. Pope John Paul II, " 'Stand Up' For Human Life," *Origins: NC Documentary Service* 9.18 (October 18, 1979) 279.
36. McCormick, *How Brave a New World?, p. 328.*
37. On this see the excellent treatment of the Genesis accounts given by Edward Schillebeeckx, *Marriage: Human Reality and Saving Mystery* New York: Sheed and Ward, 1965), vol. 1, ch. 1. See also the marvelous set of addresses given by Pope John Paul II from September 25, 1979 to April 8, 1980 probing these accounts. These addresses are printed in the English edition of *Osservatore Romano.*

38. Here see Schillebeeckx' discussion of the New Testament teaching on Marriage, especially the teaching in 1 Corinthians 7, *Marriage,* vol. 2, chs. 1 and 2.
39. International Theological Commission, "Propositions on the Doctrine of Christian Marriage," 3.4, *Origins: NC Documentary Service* (September 22, 1978) 235-239.
40. *Gaudium et Spes,* n. 48.
41. On this see Council of Florence, *Enchiridion Symbolorum,* ed. Henricus Denzinger and Adolphus Schönmetzer (33 ed. Rome: Herder, 1963), n. 1327. See also Pope Pius XI, *Casti Connubii,* par. 6.
42. The Protestant theologian Helmut Thielicke has put this quite well: "Not uniqueness establishes the marriage, but marriage establishes the uniqueness." See his *The Ethics of Sex* (New York: Harper and Row, 1963), p. 95.
43. The act of matrimonial consent is not an act concerning property rights. As Aquinas put it, the act of matrimonial consent is precisely that, a consent to marriage and to all that marriage involves, and it involves a life of friendship between husband and wife, a friendship that is to be, next to the friendship between the individual and God, the most intimate of friendships (cf. *In IV Sent*. d. 26, 2, on matrimonial consent and *Summa Contra Gentiles* 3, 123, on the greatness of conjugal friendship).
44. *Gaudium et Spes,* n. 48.
45. On this see Josef Pieper, *About Love* (Chicago: Franciscan Herald Press, 1974), pp. 50-52; Dietrich von Hildebrand, *Man and Woman* (Chicago: Franciscan Herald Press, 1968).
46. *Gaudium et Spes,* n. 49.
47. Pieper, *About Love,* p. 51.
48. An interesting and important discussion of this subject is provided by George Gilder, *Sexual Suicide* (New York: Quadrangle Books, 1973), ch. 2.
49. *Gaudium et Spes,* nn. 48, 50.
50. Man and woman become husband and wife in and through the act of matrimonial consent; the marital act does not make them to be husband and wife; it *is* marital *because* they already are husband and wife. They can freely choose not to engage in marital acts, and some people do make this choice.
51. It is important to emphasize this matter. I believe that the marital act is indeed an act that perfects and uniquely manifests married love, but it is by no means exhaustive of that love nor is it necessarily its greatest expression. There is a time for embracing, and there is a time not to embrace, and at times husband and wife can show greater love for one another by choosing not to embrace coitally than by choosing to do so.
52. See St. Thomas Aquinas, *Summa Theologiae,* 3, Supplement, q. 48, a. 1.
53. *Gaudium et Spes,* n. 49.
54. Pope Paul VI, *Humanae Vitae,* n. 11.
55. Pope John Paul II, "Revelation and Discovery of the Nuptial Meaning of the Body," Address of January 9, 1980, in *Osservatore Romano,* English ed., N. 2 (615) (January 14, 1980).
56. On this see John Kippley, *Birth Control and the Marriage Covenant*

(Collegeville, Minn.: The Liturgical Press, 1976), pp. 105-113; Dietrich von Hildebrand, *In Defense of Purity* (Chicago: Franciscan Herald Press, 1968), pp. 54-76; Mary Rosera Joyce, *Love Responds to Life* (Kenosha, Wi.: Prow Press, 1970), pp. 8-26.

57. See Robert Joyce for a stimulating and provocative discussion of maleness as a mode of sexuality with a thrust toward giving in a receiving sort of way and femaleness as a mode of sexuality with a thrust toward receiving in a giving sort of way, in his *Human Sexual Ecology* (Washington: University Publications, 1980).
58. Here it is important to stress again that what makes marriage to be marriage is the irrevocable act of free consent establishing the uniqueness of the spouses for one another. When persons who have not made themselves spouses by this free and irrevocable act of personal consent engage in coition, they cannot express marital love precisely because they have not made each other irreplaceable, nonsubstitutable persons; each remains *in principle* a replaceable and substitutable individual, not an irreplaceable and substitutable person.
59. For a development of this see my *Sex, Marriage, and Chastity,* ch. 3.
60. See, for instance, Robert and Anna Francoeur's advocacy of such creative adultery in their "The Technology of Man-Made Sex," in *The Future of Sexual Relations* (Englewood Cliffs, N.J.: Prentice-Hall, 1973). See also the views set forth by Anthony Kosnik et al., *Human Sexuality: New Directions in American Catholic Thought* (New York: Paulist Press, 1977), pp. 148-149.
61. For instance, Joseph F. Fletcher in his *The Ethics of Genetic Control.*
62. Here it is very important to call to mind the revealing, if inadvertent, remark made by Dr. Robert Edwards (one of the doctors involved in the laboratory generation of Louise Brown by in vitro fertilization): "The last time I saw *her, she* was just eight cells in a test tube. *She* was beautiful *then,* and she's still beautiful *now" (Science Digest,* October, 1978, 9; emphasis added). Surely this is eloquent tetimony that human life begins at fertilization.
63. I have been informed that this may be a very realistic possibility by Dr. Joseph Ricotta, an eminent Catholic gynecologist in Buffalo, New York.
64. I wish to observe here that should the procedure become possible, one would first have to meet conditions regarding risks to the child conceived. There would not, in this instance, be any "experimentation" being done on the human life in the laboratory; nevertheless, studies in animals should be carried out to see whether this procedure might itself cause any harm to progeny.

INDEX